Castor Oil Therapy Guide for Beginners

Understanding the Benefits of Castor Oil Therapy

By

Aulay Bryce

Copyright@2023

Table of Contents

4

CHAPTER 1

Introduction

1.1 What is Castor Oil Therapy

Castor Oil Therapy, also known as Castor Oil Packs, is a time-tested natural healing method that involves the external application of castor oil to the body, typically in a specific area of concern. This therapeutic approach has a rich history dating back centuries, with origins in ancient India, Egypt, and traditional Chinese medicine. Castor Oil Therapy is rooted in the belief that castor oil, derived from the castor bean (Ricinus communis), possesses potent healing properties that can support and enhance the body's natural processes of detoxification, relaxation, and healing.

The central element of Castor Oil Therapy is the castor oil pack, which is a cloth soaked in castor oil and applied to the skin, often over an organ or area experiencing discomfort or imbalance. This cloth is typically covered with a plastic sheet or wrap, followed by a heating pad or hot water bottle to maintain warmth. The therapy usually involves wearing the pack for an extended period, often ranging from 30 minutes to a few hours, allowing the beneficial components of castor oil to penetrate the skin and reach the underlying tissues.

Castor Oil Therapy is rooted in several key principles:

- **Detoxification:** Castor oil is believed to stimulate the lymphatic system and help the body eliminate toxins, waste, and excess fluids.

- **Pain Relief:** It is thought to alleviate pain and inflammation by promoting relaxation of the targeted area and improving circulation.

- **Improved Digestion:** Castor Oil Packs applied to the abdomen may support digestive health by soothing discomfort, reducing bloating, and aiding in the elimination of waste.

- **Skin Care:** The therapy is used for promoting healthy skin by reducing blemishes, moisturizing, and rejuvenating the complexion.

- **Relaxation:** The process of applying a castor oil pack can be deeply relaxing, aiding in stress reduction and enhancing overall well-being.

1.2 Benefits of Castor Oil Therapy

Castor Oil Therapy offers a wide range of potential benefits for individuals seeking a holistic and natural approach to health and well-being. Some of the notable benefits include:

- **Pain Management:** Castor Oil Packs are often used to alleviate pain associated with conditions like muscle strains, joint discomfort, menstrual cramps, and headaches. The application of heat and castor oil is believed to help relax tense muscles and reduce inflammation.

- **Detoxification:** Castor Oil Therapy is considered an effective method for supporting the body's detoxification process. By improving lymphatic circulation and encouraging the removal of waste and toxins, it may help individuals feel rejuvenated and more energized.

- **Digestive Health:** Applying castor oil packs to the abdomen is believed to aid digestion by promoting bowel regularity, reducing bloating, and relieving discomfort associated with conditions like irritable bowel syndrome (IBS).

- **Skin Care:** Castor oil is rich in fatty acids and antioxidants, making it a popular choice for promoting healthy and radiant skin. Regular use of castor oil packs on the face can help reduce blemishes, hydrate the skin, and diminish the signs of aging.

- **Stress Reduction:** The process of applying a castor oil pack, often accompanied by relaxation techniques, can have a calming effect, reducing stress and promoting a sense of well-being.

It's important to note that while Castor Oil Therapy has been embraced by many for its potential benefits, it is essential to consult with a healthcare professional before beginning any new therapeutic regimen, especially if you have pre-existing medical conditions or are pregnant. Additionally, individual responses to Castor Oil Therapy may vary, and its effectiveness can depend on various factors such as the quality of castor oil used and the consistency of application. Always proceed with caution and consider seeking guidance from a qualified healthcare provider to ensure your safety and well-being.

CHAPTER 2

Getting Started with Castor Oil

2.1 Types of Castor Oil

Castor oil comes in several variations, each with its unique characteristics and applications. Understanding these types is essential for effective Castor Oil Therapy. Here are the most common types:

- **Cold-Pressed Castor Oil:** This is the purest and most preferred form of castor oil for therapy. It is obtained by pressing castor beans without applying heat. Cold-pressed castor oil retains more of its natural nutrients and is typically lighter in color. It's the ideal choice for therapeutic applications due to its purity and effectiveness.

- **Jamaican Black Castor Oil (JBCO):** JBCO is a popular variant known for its dark color and distinct roasted scent. It is produced differently from cold-pressed castor oil, where the castor beans are roasted before pressing. JBCO is often used for hair and scalp treatments and is believed to promote hair growth and nourish the scalp.

- **Hydrogenated Castor Oil:** This type of castor oil is used in various industrial applications and is not suitable for Castor Oil Therapy. It has undergone a hydrogenation process, altering its chemical composition, and is not safe for topical application.

- **Deodorized Castor Oil:**
  Deodorized castor oil has had its natural scent removed and is typically used in cosmetic and skincare products where the natural aroma of castor oil may be undesirable. It is not commonly used in Castor Oil Therapy due to the removal of its natural components.

2.2 Choosing the Right Castor Oil

Selecting the right castor oil is crucial for a successful Castor Oil Therapy experience. Here are some tips to help you make the right choice:

- **Look for Cold-Pressed Castor Oil:** When engaging in Castor Oil Therapy, opt for cold-pressed castor oil as it is the most pure and suitable choice. Ensure the label specifies "cold-pressed" to guarantee its quality.

- **Consider Organic Options:** Organic castor oil is sourced from castor beans that are grown without the use of synthetic pesticides and chemicals. Choosing organic castor oil can minimize your exposure to potentially harmful residues.

- **Check for Additives:** Some castor oil products may contain additives or preservatives. Read the product label carefully to ensure it is free from unnecessary chemicals or synthetic ingredients.

- **Assess the Packaging:** Castor oil is light-sensitive and can degrade when exposed to sunlight. Choose castor oil that is packaged in dark, opaque bottles to protect it from light. This ensures the oil's longevity and effectiveness.

- **Consult Healthcare Professionals:** If you have specific health concerns or medical conditions, it's advisable to consult with a healthcare professional or a naturopathic practitioner. They can provide guidance on the type of castor oil that is most suitable for your individual needs.

By considering these factors and choosing the right type of castor oil, you can maximize the effectiveness and safety of your Castor Oil Therapy. Remember that the quality of the castor oil you use plays a significant role in achieving the desired therapeutic results, so it's worth investing in a high-quality product.

2.3 Supplies and Equipment

Before you begin Castor Oil Therapy, it's important to gather the necessary supplies and equipment to ensure a comfortable and effective experience. Here's a list of items you will need:

1. **High-Quality Castor Oil:** As discussed in the previous

section, choose cold-pressed castor oil for therapeutic purposes. Ensure it is pure and free from additives.

2. **Flannel Cloth or Wool Flannel:** You'll need a piece of flannel or wool flannel large enough to cover the area you intend to treat. It should be approximately the size of a small towel or cloth. Flannel is commonly used due to its ability to absorb and hold the castor oil effectively.

3. **Plastic Sheet or Wrap:** To prevent the castor oil from leaking or staining your clothing or bedding, you'll need a plastic sheet or plastic wrap. This should be larger than the flannel cloth.

4. **Heating Pad or Hot Water Bottle:** A heating pad or hot water bottle is used to provide gentle warmth to the castor oil pack. It's essential for the absorption of castor oil into the skin and underlying tissues. Make sure the heating pad or bottle is in good working condition and safe to use.

5. **Old Clothing or Towel:** Wear old clothing or use a towel to protect your clothing and bedding from potential oil stains. Castor oil can be challenging to remove from fabric, so it's best to use something you don't mind getting oil on.

6. **Large Plastic Bag or Plastic Wrap Roll:** After use, store the castor oil pack and flannel in a

large plastic bag or wrap it in plastic wrap. This prevents the pack from drying out and allows you to reuse it multiple times.

7. **Tape or Bandage:** You may need tape or a bandage to secure the castor oil pack in place, especially if you plan to move around while using it.

8. **Timer or Clock:** It's essential to keep track of the duration of the therapy. A timer or a clock with a second hand can help you ensure that you use the pack for the recommended amount of time.

9. **Comfortable and Relaxing Space:** Find a quiet and comfortable space where you can relax during the therapy

session. This may include a comfortable chair, couch, or a bed.

10. **Old Towels or Washcloths:** Keep some old towels or washcloths nearby for cleaning up any excess castor oil on your skin after removing the pack.

11. **Optional Aromatherapy:** Some individuals choose to enhance the relaxation aspect of Castor Oil Therapy with aromatherapy. You can use essential oils in a diffuser to create a calming atmosphere.

Assemble these supplies and equipment before you start Castor Oil Therapy to ensure a smooth and stress-free experience. Being well-prepared not only makes the process more comfortable but also maximizes the potential benefits of this natural healing method.

CHAPTER 3
Understanding Castor Oil Packs

3.1 What Are Castor Oil Packs

Castor Oil Packs are a central component of Castor Oil Therapy and are widely used for their potential therapeutic benefits. A Castor Oil Pack is a simple yet effective external application of castor oil to the skin, typically over a specific area of concern or discomfort. Here's a breakdown of what Castor Oil Packs entail:

- **Materials**: A Castor Oil Pack consists of several materials, primarily a piece of flannel or wool flannel that has been soaked in castor oil. This cloth is typically large enough to cover the targeted area, such as the abdomen, lower back, or other body parts.

- **Application**: The castor oil-soaked cloth is placed directly on the skin over the area of interest. To prevent leakage and maintain warmth, a plastic sheet or plastic wrap is often placed over the cloth. A heating pad or hot water bottle is then applied over the plastic to gently warm the pack.

- **Duration**: Castor Oil Packs are typically worn for an extended period, usually ranging from 30 minutes to a few hours. The duration can vary depending on the individual's needs and the specific condition being addressed.

- **Frequency**: The frequency of Castor Oil Pack application also varies. Some people use them daily, while others may apply them a few times a week. The recommended frequency often depends on the purpose of the therapy and the individual's response.

- **Storage**: After each use, Castor Oil Packs should be stored in a plastic bag or wrapped in plastic wrap to prevent them from drying out. They can be reused multiple times before needing to be replaced.

3.2 How Castor Oil Packs Work

Castor Oil Packs are believed to work through several mechanisms to promote health and well-being. While the scientific evidence supporting these claims is limited, many people have reported positive outcomes from using Castor Oil Packs. Here's an overview of how they are thought to work:

- **Stimulation of Lymphatic Flow:** Castor Oil Packs are believed to enhance the circulation of lymphatic fluids. The lymphatic system is responsible for removing waste, toxins, and excess fluids from the body. By promoting lymphatic flow, Castor Oil Packs may support the body's natural detoxification processes.

- **Improvement of Blood Circulation:** The application of warmth through the heating pad or hot water bottle can help dilate blood vessels and improve blood circulation in the targeted area. This increased blood flow may aid in reducing inflammation and promoting healing.

- **Relaxation and Stress Reduction:** The process of applying a Castor Oil Pack and relaxing during the therapy session can have a calming effect. Reducing stress and promoting relaxation is believed to be an integral part of the healing process.

- **Localized Healing and Pain Relief:** Castor Oil is thought to have analgesic (pain-relieving) and anti-inflammatory properties. When applied topically, it may help alleviate discomfort and reduce inflammation in the specific area where the pack is placed.

- **Hydration and Nourishment of the Skin:** Castor oil is rich in fatty acids, which can help moisturize and nourish the skin. This is particularly beneficial when Castor Oil Packs are used for skincare applications, such as reducing blemishes and promoting healthy, radiant skin.

It's important to note that while Castor Oil Packs are well-regarded by many as a holistic therapeutic method, their effectiveness can vary from person to person. If you are considering using Castor Oil Packs, it's advisable to consult with a healthcare professional or naturopathic practitioner, especially if you have specific health concerns or conditions. They can provide guidance on the appropriate use of Castor Oil Packs based on your individual needs.

3.3 When to Use Castor Oil Packs

Castor Oil Packs can be a beneficial addition to your wellness routine, but it's important to know when to use them to maximize their effectiveness. The timing and frequency of Castor Oil Pack application can vary based on individual needs and the specific goals you want to achieve. Here are some common scenarios and

guidelines for when to use Castor Oil
Packs:

1. **For Pain and Inflammation:**
   Castor Oil Packs can be used
   when you are experiencing
   localized pain or inflammation,
   such as muscle strains, joint
   discomfort, or menstrual
   cramps. Apply the pack to the
   affected area to help alleviate
   pain and reduce inflammation.
   This can be done as needed
   when you experience
   discomfort.

2. **Digestive Issues:** If you're
   dealing with digestive
   problems, including bloating,
   constipation, or irritable bowel
   syndrome (IBS), you can use
   Castor Oil Packs on your
   abdomen. Applying them
   regularly, such as a few times a

week, may help soothe digestive discomfort and support healthy bowel movements.

3. **Detoxification:** Many individuals use Castor Oil Packs as part of a detoxification regimen. You can use them as a weekly or monthly detox ritual to help your body eliminate toxins, waste, and excess fluids. This can be particularly helpful if you've been exposed to environmental toxins or want to support your liver's detoxification functions.

4. **Skincare and Beauty:** Castor Oil Packs can be incorporated into your skincare routine. If you're looking to reduce blemishes, moisturize your skin, or rejuvenate your

complexion, use the packs on your face as part of a skincare regimen. The frequency can vary, but weekly applications are common.

5. **Menstrual Support:** For women experiencing menstrual discomfort or irregular periods, using Castor Oil Packs on the lower abdomen can provide relief. Start a few days before your period and continue through the cycle to help ease cramps and promote a healthier menstrual flow.

6. **Fertility and Reproductive Health:** Some individuals use Castor Oil Packs to support reproductive health. If you're trying to conceive or addressing fertility issues, consider using the packs on the lower

abdomen as part of your fertility support regimen. The timing may vary based on your specific situation, and it's advisable to consult with a healthcare professional.

7. **General Wellness and Stress Reduction:** Castor Oil Packs can be used as a relaxation and stress-reduction tool. Apply them when you need a moment of calm and relaxation. This can be done as often as desired to support overall well-being.

The frequency and timing of Castor Oil Pack application can be personalized based on your unique needs and goals. It's essential to listen to your body and observe how you respond to the therapy. If you have specific health concerns or are unsure about the timing, it's a good idea to consult with a healthcare professional or naturopathic practitioner for guidance tailored to your individual circumstances.

CHAPTER 4

Preparing for Castor Oil Therapy

4.1 Safety Precautions

Before you embark on Castor Oil Therapy, it's important to take certain safety precautions to ensure a safe and effective experience. Here are some key safety considerations to keep in mind:

- **Consult a Healthcare Professional:** If you have underlying health conditions, are pregnant, nursing, or taking medications, it's crucial to consult with a healthcare professional before beginning Castor Oil Therapy. They can provide guidance and determine if this therapy is appropriate for your situation.

- **Allergies and Sensitivities:** Be aware of potential allergies or sensitivities to castor oil. While allergies to castor oil are rare, they can occur. Perform a skin patch test (detailed in the next section) to check for any adverse reactions before using a Castor Oil Pack on a larger area.

- **Quality of Castor Oil:** Ensure that you are using high-quality, cold-pressed castor oil that is free from additives or contaminants. Inferior or impure oils can potentially cause adverse reactions.

- **Avoid Broken Skin:** Do not use Castor Oil Packs on broken or irritated skin, wounds, or open sores. This could lead to infection or skin irritation.

- **Heat Application Safety:** When using a heating pad or hot water bottle in conjunction with Castor Oil Packs, ensure that the temperature is not too hot. The application of excessive heat can cause burns or discomfort. Use a towel or cloth between the pack and the heating source to moderate the temperature.

- **Supervision:** If using Castor Oil Therapy on children or individuals who may have difficulty managing the therapy themselves, ensure proper

supervision to prevent
accidents or misuse.

- **Cleaning and Maintenance:**
  Regularly clean the materials
  used in Castor Oil Therapy,
  such as the flannel cloth and
  plastic sheet, to prevent mold or
  bacterial growth. Store the
  materials in a clean, dry place
  between uses.

- **Discontinue If Adverse
  Reactions Occur:** If you
  experience any adverse
  reactions, such as skin
  irritation, itching, or
  discomfort, discontinue the
  therapy and wash the affected
  area with mild soap and water.

- **Potential Discomfort:** Be
  prepared for some discomfort
  or a slight mess while using

Castor Oil Packs. Castor oil can be sticky, and the pack may feel heavy. This is normal and usually outweighed by the potential benefits.

4.2 Skin Patch Test

Performing a skin patch test is an essential step before using Castor Oil Packs, especially if you've never used castor oil on your skin. A patch test helps you identify any allergic reactions or sensitivities to castor oil. Here's how to conduct a skin patch test:

1. **Select a Small Area:** Choose a small, inconspicuous area on your skin, such as the inside of your forearm or the back of your wrist.

2. **Clean the Area:** Wash the chosen area with mild soap and water, then pat it dry.

3. **Apply a Small Amount of Castor Oil:** Apply a small amount of castor oil (just a few drops) to the selected area.

4. **Cover and Wait:** Cover the area with a clean bandage or adhesive tape to keep the castor oil in place. Leave it on for 24 hours.

5. **Observe for Reactions:** After 24 hours, carefully remove the bandage and inspect the area. Look for signs of redness, itching, swelling, or any other skin reactions.

If you experience any adverse reactions during the patch test, such as skin irritation or an allergic response, discontinue the use of castor oil and consult a healthcare professional. If no adverse reactions occur, it is generally safe to proceed with Castor Oil Therapy.

By taking these safety precautions and conducting a skin patch test, you can help ensure that Castor Oil Therapy is a safe and beneficial addition to your wellness routine.

4.3 Selecting a Suitable Area

Choosing the right area of your body for applying a Castor Oil Pack is a crucial step in the Castor Oil Therapy process. The effectiveness of the therapy can be influenced by the specific area you target. Here's how to select a suitable area:

1. **Identify the Area of Concern:** Determine the area of your body that requires attention or relief. This could be a region experiencing pain, discomfort, inflammation, or a specific condition you're addressing.

2. **Consider the Purpose:** The purpose of your Castor Oil Therapy will guide your choice of the area. For example, if you're using it for digestive support, you'll typically apply it to the abdomen. If it's for skincare, the face is the target area.

3. **Safety and Comfort:** Ensure that the chosen area is accessible and comfortable for applying the Castor Oil Pack. Avoid areas with broken or irritated skin, wounds, or open

sores, as these may become further aggravated by the therapy.

4. **Size of the Flannel Cloth:** Choose a flannel cloth that is appropriately sized to cover the selected area. The cloth should be large enough to provide adequate coverage but not so large that it becomes unwieldy.

5. **Warmth and Comfort:** Consider the practicality of applying a heating pad or hot water bottle to the area. It's essential that you can comfortably maintain the warmth of the pack while it's in place.

6. **Privacy and Relaxation:** Select a location where you can relax during the therapy

session. Castor Oil Therapy is often a calming and stress-reducing practice, so choose a space that offers privacy and comfort.

Common areas for Castor Oil Pack application include:

- **Abdomen:** The abdomen is a popular choice for addressing digestive issues, menstrual cramps, and detoxification. It's easily accessible and can be kept warm with a heating pad.

- **Lower Back:** Applying the pack to the lower back is often chosen for addressing back pain, muscle tension, or discomfort in that area.

- **Face and Neck:** Castor Oil Packs can be used for skincare benefits on the face and neck.

They can help reduce blemishes, hydrate the skin, and promote a healthy complexion.

- **Pelvic Area:** Some individuals use Castor Oil Packs on the pelvic area to support reproductive health and address issues like ovarian cysts or fertility concerns.

- **Joints and Muscles:** For joint pain or muscle discomfort in specific areas, such as the knees or shoulders, you can target those regions with Castor Oil Packs.

Ultimately, the area you choose for Castor Oil Pack application should align with your specific health goals and preferences. It's essential to feel comfortable and relaxed during the therapy, as this can contribute to its effectiveness. If you have any doubts about the suitability of the area or are unsure about the therapy's application for a particular condition, consult with a healthcare professional or a naturopathic practitioner for personalized guidance.

CHAPTER 5

Applying Castor Oil Therapy

5.1 Setting Up the Environment

Before applying Castor Oil Therapy, it's important to create a suitable environment for a comfortable and effective experience. Here's how to set up your environment:

1. **Choose a Quiet Space:** Find a quiet and peaceful area where you can relax during the therapy session. Create an atmosphere that promotes calm and stress reduction.

2. **Protect the Surface:** Lay down an old towel or cloth on the surface where you plan to lie or sit. This helps protect it from potential oil stains.

3. **Gather Supplies:** Ensure you have all the necessary supplies and equipment ready, including the Castor Oil Pack, heating pad or hot water bottle, timer, and any additional items you may need.

4. **Adjust Lighting:** Dim the lights or use soft lighting to enhance relaxation. Some individuals choose to use aromatherapy, such as essential oils in a diffuser, to create a calming atmosphere.

5. **Dress Comfortably:** Wear loose, comfortable clothing that

allows you to relax and move freely if needed. You can also wrap yourself in a cozy blanket for added comfort.

6. **Privacy:** If you prefer privacy during the therapy, find a space where you won't be disturbed. This is especially important if you want to engage in relaxation techniques during the session.

7. **Take a Few Deep Breaths:** Before starting, take a few deep breaths to center yourself and prepare for the therapy. Deep, slow breaths can help you relax and get the most out of the experience.

5.2 Applying the Pack

Here's a step-by-step guide on how to apply a Castor Oil Pack:

1. **Position Yourself:** Lie down or sit in a comfortable position. If you're using the pack on an area that requires a specific posture, ensure you're in the correct position.

2. **Place the Pack:** Lay the Castor Oil Pack, which consists of the flannel cloth soaked in castor oil, directly over the targeted area on your body. Ensure the plastic sheet or plastic wrap is underneath to prevent oil from seeping through.

3. **Add Heat:** Place the heating pad or hot water bottle on top of the flannel cloth. Ensure it's set to a comfortable and safe

temperature. You may want to cover the heating pad with a towel to moderate the heat.

4. **Secure in Place (Optional):** If you need to move around during the therapy or feel more secure with the pack in place, you can use tape or a bandage to secure it.

5. **Relax and Breathe:** Once the pack is in place and the heat is applied, focus on relaxation. You can close your eyes, take deep breaths, meditate, or engage in any relaxation techniques that work for you.

6. **Set a Timer:** Use a timer or clock to keep track of the duration of the therapy. The recommended duration can vary based on your goals and

the specific area you are
targeting.

5.3 Duration and Frequency

The duration and frequency of Castor
Oil Therapy can vary depending on
your goals and individual needs. Here
are some general guidelines:

- **Duration:** The duration of a
  Castor Oil Pack session
  typically ranges from 30
  minutes to a few hours. Shorter
  sessions may be appropriate for
  daily use, while longer sessions
  might be reserved for less
  frequent applications.

- **Frequency:** The frequency of
  Castor Oil Pack application can
  also vary:

- **For pain and inflammation:** You can use the pack as needed whenever you experience discomfort.

- **For digestive support:** A few times a week is common for addressing digestive issues.

- **For detoxification:** You can incorporate Castor Oil Packs into your detox regimen, which may be done weekly or monthly.

- **For skincare:** Using the pack once a week can be suitable for maintaining healthy skin.

It's important to listen to your body and assess how you respond to Castor Oil Therapy. If you have specific health concerns or are unsure about the appropriate duration and frequency, consult with a healthcare professional or naturopathic practitioner. They can provide personalized guidance tailored to your unique needs and goals.

CHAPTER 6

Health and Wellness Applications

6.1 Relieving Pain and Inflammation

Castor Oil Therapy can be used to relieve pain and inflammation in various parts of the body. It's especially helpful for addressing localized discomfort and promoting relaxation. Here's how it can be applied for pain relief and inflammation reduction:

- **Muscle Pain and Tension:** Apply a Castor Oil Pack to the area with muscle pain or tension. The heat and castor oil may help relax muscles and reduce pain.

- **Joint Discomfort:** Use the pack on joints, such as knees or shoulders, to alleviate joint discomfort and improve flexibility.

- **Menstrual Cramps:** Applying a pack to the lower abdomen can help relieve menstrual cramps and promote a healthier menstrual flow.

- **Back Pain:** The lower back is a common area for addressing back pain. The pack can provide relief by reducing inflammation and relaxing the affected muscles.

6.2 Digestive Health

Castor Oil Packs are often used to support digestive health. Here's how they can be beneficial in this context:

- **Irritable Bowel Syndrome (IBS):** Applying a Castor Oil Pack to the abdomen may help soothe discomfort and support digestive regularity in individuals with IBS.

- **Bloating:** The therapy can reduce bloating and gas by improving circulation and helping the digestive system function more effectively.

- **Constipation:** Castor Oil Packs may aid in alleviating constipation by promoting healthy bowel movements.

6.3 Skin Care and Beauty

Castor Oil Packs can be incorporated into skincare and beauty routines to promote healthy, radiant skin. Here's how they can be used for skincare and beauty purposes:

- **Reducing Blemishes:** Apply Castor Oil Packs to the face to reduce blemishes, such as acne and pimples. The oil's antibacterial properties can help cleanse the skin.

- **Hydration:** Castor oil is rich in fatty acids, which can moisturize the skin and prevent dryness.

- **Anti-Aging:** Regular use of Castor Oil Packs on the face can help reduce the signs of aging, such as fine lines and wrinkles, by promoting collagen production and skin elasticity.

6.4 Detoxification

Castor Oil Therapy is often used as part of detoxification regimens. Here's how it can support detoxification:

- **Lymphatic System:** Castor Oil Packs are believed to stimulate the lymphatic system, promoting the removal of toxins, waste, and excess fluids from the body.

- **Liver Support:** The therapy is thought to aid the liver in its detoxification processes by reducing congestion and promoting healthy liver function.

- **Environmental Toxins:** Castor Oil Packs can be particularly helpful in cases of potential exposure to environmental toxins. They can assist in clearing toxins from the body.

It's important to note that while Castor Oil Therapy has been embraced for its potential benefits in these areas, its effectiveness can vary from person to person. Individual responses depend on various factors, including the quality of castor oil used, the consistency of application, and overall health. If you are considering Castor Oil Therapy for specific health or wellness goals, consult with a healthcare professional or a naturopathic practitioner for guidance tailored to your unique needs.

CHAPTER 7

Castor Oil Therapy for Specific Conditions

7.1 Joint and Muscle Pain

Castor Oil Therapy can be particularly beneficial for addressing joint and muscle pain. The soothing properties of castor oil and the therapeutic benefits of the therapy make it a valuable option for natural pain relief. Here's how to apply Castor Oil Therapy for joint and muscle pain:

1. **Materials Needed:** Gather the necessary materials, including high-quality cold-pressed castor oil, a piece of flannel cloth or

wool flannel, plastic sheet or plastic wrap, a heating pad or hot water bottle, old clothing or a towel, and a timer.

2. **Prepare the Pack:** Cut the flannel cloth to the appropriate size to cover the painful joint or muscle. Soak the cloth in castor oil and wring out any excess. Place the cloth on a plastic sheet.

3. **Apply the Pack:** Lay the soaked cloth on the painful area. Place the plastic sheet or plastic wrap on top of the cloth to prevent oil from leaking. Then, use the heating pad or hot water bottle on top to provide gentle warmth to the pack.

4. **Secure the Pack (Optional):** If you need to move around during the therapy, use tape or a bandage to secure the pack in place.

5. **Relax and Time It:** Lie down or sit comfortably, and set a timer for the recommended duration, typically 30 minutes to an hour. The warmth and castor oil can help reduce inflammation and alleviate pain in the targeted area.

6. **Frequency:** You can use Castor Oil Packs for joint and muscle pain as needed. This may involve daily applications for acute pain or a few times a week for chronic discomfort.

7. **Consult a Professional:** If you have a specific joint or muscle

condition, consider consulting with a healthcare professional or physical therapist for guidance on the appropriate use of Castor Oil Therapy for your situation.

Castor Oil Therapy for joint and muscle pain is an excellent complement to other pain management strategies and physical therapies. It can provide relief, promote relaxation, and support overall wellness, but it's important to use it as part of a comprehensive approach to managing pain and discomfort.

7.2 Hair and Scalp Conditions

Castor Oil Therapy can be used to address a variety of hair and scalp conditions. Castor oil is renowned for its potential benefits in promoting healthy hair and alleviating common hair and scalp issues. Here's how to use Castor Oil Therapy for hair and scalp conditions:

1. **Materials Needed:** To get started, you'll require high-quality cold-pressed castor oil, an old T-shirt or a towel, a plastic shower cap, a wide-tooth comb, and a timer.

2. **Prepare the Castor Oil Treatment:**

    - Warm a small amount of castor oil by placing it in

a heatproof container and immersing it in hot water for a few minutes. Ensure it's comfortably warm, not hot.

3. **Application:** Follow these steps for a hair and scalp treatment:

   - Part your hair into sections and apply the warmed castor oil to your scalp using your fingertips. Massage gently to ensure the oil is evenly distributed.

   - Dip a wide-tooth comb into the oil and comb through your hair to distribute it along the strands.

- Pile your hair on top of your head and cover it with a plastic shower cap. This helps to retain heat and moisture.

4. **Duration:** Leave the Castor Oil Therapy treatment on your hair and scalp for at least 30 minutes to an hour. For a more intensive treatment, you can leave it on overnight, but be sure to protect your pillow with an old towel or cloth.

5. **Rinse and Shampoo:** After the recommended duration, wash your hair thoroughly with a mild shampoo. You may need to shampoo twice to remove all the oil.

6. **Frequency:** For general hair and scalp health, you can use

Castor Oil Therapy once a week. If you're targeting a specific issue, such as dandruff or hair thinning, consult a healthcare professional or dermatologist for personalized guidance on the frequency of application.

7. **Hair Growth:** Many people use Castor Oil Therapy to promote hair growth. While there is limited scientific evidence to support this, some individuals massage castor oil into their scalp regularly to potentially encourage hair growth. Be patient, as results may take time.

8. **Hair and Scalp Issues:** Castor oil can also be used to address issues like dandruff, dry scalp, and split ends. Regular

applications may help improve the condition of your hair and scalp.

Individual results may vary, and the effectiveness of Castor Oil Therapy for hair and scalp conditions can depend on factors such as the quality of castor oil, the specific issue you're addressing, and your consistency in using the therapy. If you have persistent hair or scalp concerns, it's advisable to consult with a dermatologist or hair care specialist for a tailored treatment plan.

CHAPTER 8

Frequently Asked Questions

8.1 Common Concerns

In the course of using Castor Oil Therapy, you may encounter some common concerns or questions. Here are a few of them, along with potential solutions:

1. Oil Stains: Castor oil can be challenging to remove from fabric. To prevent oil stains, use old clothing or towels during therapy. If you do get oil on fabric, act quickly to blot with a paper towel, then use a mixture of dish soap and water to clean the stain.

2. Skin Irritation: While rare, some people may experience skin irritation or an allergic reaction. Conduct a skin patch test before using Castor Oil Packs, and if irritation occurs, discontinue use.

3. Leaking: To prevent oil from leaking through the flannel cloth, ensure that the cloth is not oversaturated with oil. You can also use additional plastic wrap or plastic sheeting for added protection.

4. Maintaining Warmth: If the heating pad or hot water bottle doesn't maintain a consistent temperature, use a towel or cloth between the pack and the heating source to moderate the heat.

5. Dry Cloth: Over time, the flannel cloth may dry out between uses. Reapply a small amount of castor oil before each use to keep the cloth adequately moist.

6. Frequent Use: While Castor Oil Therapy can be used frequently for certain conditions, it's essential not to overuse it. Consult with a healthcare professional for guidance on the appropriate frequency based on your specific needs.

8.2 Troubleshooting

If you encounter issues or have concerns while using Castor Oil Therapy, consider the following troubleshooting tips:

1. Skin Sensitivity: If you have sensitive skin or experience skin irritation, use a thinner layer of castor oil on the flannel cloth during the next application. If the issue persists, consider using a different carrier oil, such as coconut oil, which may be gentler on the skin.

2. Leaking or Messiness: To minimize leaks, ensure the flannel cloth is not oversaturated. Wring out any excess oil before applying the pack. Additionally, be mindful of your body position during the therapy to prevent unnecessary movement that can lead to spills.

3. Discomfort from Heat: If the heating pad or hot water bottle feels too hot or uncomfortable, place a towel or cloth between the pack and the heating source to regulate the temperature. It's important to maintain warmth without causing discomfort.

4. Infrequent Results: If you don't see the desired results after using Castor Oil Therapy, it may be necessary to adjust the duration, frequency, or specific area you are targeting. Consult with a healthcare professional for personalized advice and assessment.

5. Quality of Castor Oil: Ensure you are using high-quality, cold-pressed castor oil. The effectiveness of the therapy is closely tied to the quality of the oil.

6. Consult a Healthcare Professional: If you encounter persistent issues or have specific health concerns, don't hesitate to consult with a healthcare professional or naturopathic practitioner. They can provide personalized guidance and address any complications you may be facing.

Castor Oil Therapy can be an excellent addition to your wellness routine, but like any holistic approach, it may require some adjustments and troubleshooting to optimize its benefits for your specific needs. Consulting with a healthcare professional can help you navigate any challenges or concerns effectively.